Treatment by Massage: its mode of application and effects

Douglas Graham

Treatment by Massage
its Mode of Application and Effects

LM Publishers

The Mode of Application and Effects of the Massage

"Massage" from the Greek *masso* (I knead or handle), is a term now generally accepted to signify a group of procedures which are usually done with the hands, such as friction, kneading, manipulating, rolling, and percussing of the external tissues of the body, either with some curative, palliative, or hygienic object in view. Its application should in many instances be combined with passive, resistive, or assistive movements, and these are often spoken of as the so-called Swedish movement-cure. There is, however, an increasing tendency on the part of scientific men to have the word "massage" embrace all these varied forms of manual therapeutics, for the reason that the word "cure," attached to any form of treatment whatsoever, cannot always be applicable, inasmuch as there are many maladies that preclude the possibility of recovery and yet admit of amelioration. Hence the. word "cure" may lead people to expect too much; and, on the other hand, the use of the word "rubbing" in place of "massage" 1 tends to undervalue the application and benefit of the latter, for it is but natural to suppose that all kinds of rubbing are alike, differing only in the amount of force used.

According to the requirements of individual cases, massage may be o primary importance or of secondary importance, of no use at all, or even injurious. Concerning the extent of its usefulness, it may with safety be said that, at tolerably definite stages in one or more classes of affections in every special and general department of medicine, evidence can be found that it has proved either directly or indirectly beneficial, or led to recovery, sometimes when other means had been but slowly operative, or apparently had failed altogether. In view of these facts, it need hardly be said that those who would properly understand and apply massage should be familiar with its past and present literature; they should also be familiar not only with the natural history of the maladies in which massage may be applied when left to themselves, but also with the course of these affections when treated in the usual approved methods, so that improvements or relapses may be referred to their proper causes. Moreover, they should know something about the methods of others who have any claim to respectability in their manner of applying massage, so as to compare them with their own. And yet all these qualifications may fail if the operator has not in addition abundance of time, patience, strength, and skill, acquired by long and intelligent experience. Measured by these requirements, I fear that good *masseurs* (manipulators) are scarce. Dr. E. C. Seguin, in the "Archives of Medicine" for April, 1881, says, that even in New York there are few manipulators who can be trusted to do massage well. Massage may be studied as a science, but it has, like everything else in medicine and surgery, to be practiced as an art. Those who have a natural tact, talent, and liking for massage, united with soft, elastic, and strong hands, and physical endurance to use them, may be as useful artists in this department of the healing art as in others. It has been well said that those who do massage should be tender and gentle, yet strong and enduring. These are qualities that are rarely found combined in manipulators. It is a very common mistake to suppose that those who are of a remarkably healthy, ruddy appearance, plethoric and fat, are the best fitted to do massage. Such people require a great deal of exercise in the open air for the proper oxygenation of their blood, and confining, indoor work, like massage, they soon find to be tedious and irksome. Besides, the stooping attitude and varying positions so often necessary while doing this sort of work soon put them out of breath; and thus, while suffering from their ignorance and awkwardness, they fancy they are imparting "magnetism" to their patients at their own expense. Better that the manipulators should be rather thin, though if of too spare a habit their hands will not be sufficiently strong and muscular and their tissues generally will lack that firmness necessary for prolonged endurance.

One of the best German medical reviews, "Schmidt's Jahrbücher," in an extensive report on massage, thus indicates the esteem in which this treatment is held by many eminent physicians and surgeons of Europe: "It is but recently that massage has gained an extensive scientific consideration, since it has passed out of the hands of rough and ignorant empirics into those of educated physicians; and upon the results of recent scientific investigations it has been cultivated into an improved therapeutical system, and has won for itself in its entirety the merit of having become a special branch of the art of medicine." Professor Billroth, one of the most eminent surgeons of Germany, in a lecture on this subject published in the "Wiener med. Wochen.," No. 45, 1875, says: "I can only agree with my colleagues, Langenbeck and Esmarch, that massage in suitable cases deserves more attention than has fallen to its lot in the course of the past ten years in Germany. . . . As practice in the manipulations, time, perseverance, and personal interest in the matter are necessary, and these one cannot bestow who interests himself much in medicine and surgery, I have turned over to my old experienced surgical assistant suitable cases for massage, and he has already obtained a series of results both favorable and surprising, and far exceeding my expectations of this method of treatment." Previous to the past fifteen years the French physicians took more interest in massage than any others, but of late they have almost entirely laid it aside. With their waning interest the Scandinavians and Germans have taken up the subject with renewed zeal, and from time to time furnish instructive accounts of their experiments, successes, and failures.

How is massage regarded, and what is its condition, in the United States? Except among very few—epicures in this matter, if one may so speak—there is as yet but little evidence of a desire to place massage, and those who do it, on their merits alone, irrespective of the policy of employing persons who are only rubbing-machines, or of tolerating obnoxious individuals so long as the poor patients' minds are satisfied. This is too often the case, and then massage is said to have failed and valuable time is lost, when, if it had been properly applied, it might have been successful; or, on the other hand, perhaps it should have been omitted and other remedies employed. The writer of this, in a recent paper on the "History of Massage," has said: "In almost every city of the United States, and indeed of the whole civilized world, there may be found individuals claiming mysterious and magical powers of curing disease, setting bones, and relieving pain by the immediate application of their hands. Some of these boldly assert that their art is a gift from Heaven, due to some unknown power which they call magnetism, while others designate it by some peculiar word ending with *pathy* or *cure,* and it is astonishing how much credit they get for their supposed genius by many of the most learned people." Let a fisherman forsake his boat, or a blacksmith his anvil, or a carpenter his bench, or a shoe-maker his shop, and proclaim that he has made the wonderful discovery that he is full of magnetism and can cure all diseases, and, be he ever so ignorant and uncouth, he is likely to have, in a remarkably short space of time, a large *clientèle* of educated gentlemen and refined ladies. It is not meant to imply that the previous occupation of such people is at all to their discredit, but, were they capable of giving a rational explanation of their doings, the halo of mystery would be removed from around them, and their prestige and patronage would suffer a sudden decline.

In Boston and Philadelphia, and perhaps in other cities as well, efforts have been made by physicians, who are thoroughly familiar with massage, to instruct intelligent nurses and others how to apply it, and at the training-schools for nurses the pupils receive some general instruction in the matter. In this way something has been accomplished to bring massage within the rules and regulations of common sense and rational therapeutics. But still there is great room for improvement even in this direction, for it is but too often the case that after one or two persons are specially trained to do massage they are requested to give instruction to some of the pupils at the schools for nurses, and to others, a few of whom, after having received some general desultory lessons, are in turn delegated or relegated to teach others. and so on, until, by the time massage reaches the needy patients, there is often little left of it but the name. Hence it is not to be wondered at that many a shrewd, superannuated auntie, and others who are out of a job, having learned the meaning of the word massage, immediately have it printed on their cards, and keep on with their "rubbin'" just as they always have done.

The vaguest generalities exist as to the manner of doing massage, even among the best authors on the subject, and, after having studied and tried the methods of all, the writer proposes to briefly formulate, as much as space will permit of, what he has found to be of value, without having adopted the methods of any in particular. By so doing it is hoped that some will be able to judge whether those employed to do massage know anything about it or not, or whether it would not be as well to employ one of their own domestics for ordinary rubbing, the advantages of which are not to be despised. At any rate, from the description which follows, I trust that not a few intelligent friends of chronic invalids, who are beyond the reach of the professional manipulator, will be enabled to apply massage so as to afford even greater relief and comfort than can be gained from many of those whom the ignorance of the community on this subject alone tolerates as experts.

The multiform subdivisions under which the various procedures of massage have been described can all be grouped under four different heads, viz., friction, percussion, pressure, and movement. Malaxation, manipulation, deep-rubbing, kneading, or massage, properly so called, is to be considered as a combination of the last two. Each and all of these may be gentle, moderate, or vigorous, according to the requirements of the case and the physical qualities of the operators. Some

18

general remarks here will save repetition: 1. All of the single or combined procedures should be begun moderately, gradually increased in force and frequency to their fullest extent desirable, and should end gradually as begun. 2. The greatest extent of surface of the fingers and hands of the operator consistent with ease and efficacy of movement should be adapted to the surface worked upon, in order that no' time be lost by working with the ends of the fingers or one portion of the hands when all the rest might be occupied. 3. The patient should be placed in as easy and comfortable a position as possible, in a well-ventilated room at a temperature of about 70° Fahr. 4. What constitutes the dose of massage is to be determined by the force and frequency of the manipulations and the length of time during which they are employed. A good manipulator will do more in fifteen minutes than a poor one will in an hour, just as an old machanic working deliberately will accomplish more than an inexperienced one working furiously. Friction has been described as rectilinear, vertical, transverse or horizontal, and circular. It has been stated, and very properly, that rectilinear friction should always be used in an upward direction, from the extremities to the trunk, so to favor and not retard the venous and lymphatic currents. But a slight deviation from this method I have found to be more advantageous, for though in almost every case the upward strokes of the friction should be the stronger, vet the returning or downward movement may with benefit lightly graze the surface, imparting a soothing influence, without being so vigorous as to retard the circulation, and thus a saving of time and effort will be gained. The manner in which a carpenter uses his plane represents this forward-and-return movement very well.

Transverse friction, or friction at right angles to the long axis of a limb, is a very ungraceful and awkward procedure. It has been introduced on theoretical considerations alone, and may with safety be laid aside, for the method already spoken of, together with circular friction, will do all and a great deal more than rubbing crosswise on a limb can do. A convenient extent of territory, to begin with, is from the ends of the fingers to the wrist, each stroke being of this length, the returning stroke being light, without raising the hand. The rapidity of these double strokes may be from one hundred to one hundred and fifty a minute. The whole palmar surface of the fingers should be employed, and in such a manner that they will fit into the depressions formed by the approximation of the phalang and metacarpal bones. The heel of the hand should be used for especially vigorous friction of the palm, as well as for the sole of the foot. From the wrist to the elbow, and from the elbow to the shoulder, are separately convenient extents of surface, and here not only straight-line friction, extending from one joint to the other, may be used, but also circular friction. The form of the latter which I have found most serviceable is in that of an oval, both hands moving at the same time, the one ascending as the other descends, at the rate of one hundred and twenty-five to two hundred and fifty each a minute, or two hundred and fifty to five hundred with both hands, each stroke reaching from joint to joint, the upward stroke being carefully kept within the limits of chafing the skin. These observations apply to the lower limbs also, but, as they are larger than the arms, the posterior and lateral aspects, from ankle to knee, will be a convenient territory, while the anterior and lateral aspects will be another for thorough and efficacious friction. The same systematic division of surface may be made above the knees as below, the number of strokes below will vary from one hundred to one hundred and sixty with each hand; above, from seventy-five to one hundred each. From the base of the skull to the spine of the scapula forms another region naturally well bounded for downward and outward semicircular friction, and from the spine of the scapula to the base of the sacrum and crest of the ilium forms another surface over which one hand can sweep, while the other works toward it from the insertion to the origin of the glutei, at an average rate of sixty or seventy-five a minute with each hand for a person of medium size. It will be observed that on the back and thighs the strokes are not so rapid as on the other parts mentioned, for the reason that the skin is here thicker and coarser, in consequence of which the hand cannot glide

23

so easily, and the larger muscles beneath can well bear stronger pressure; besides, the strokes are somewhat longer, all of which require an increased expenditure of time. The chest should be done from the insertion to the origin of the pectoral muscles, and the abdomen from the right iliac fossa in the direction of the ascending, transverse and descending colon. But here friction is seldom necessary, for the procedure about to be considered accomplishes all that friction can do, and a great deal more in this region. The force used in doing friction is often much greater than is necessary, for it is only intended to act upon the skin, and there are better ways of acting upon the tissues beneath it. If redness and irritation be looked upon as a measure of the beneficial effects of friction upon the skin, then a coarse towel, a hair mitten, or a brush would answer for this purpose a great deal better than the hand alone.

The most important, agreeable, and efficacious procedure of massage has been variously designated as manipulation, kneading, deep rubbing, or massage properly so called, in contradistinction to the more superficial method spoken of above. This is done by adapting as much as possible of the fingers and hands to the parts to be thus treated, and, without allowing them to slip on the skin, the tissues beneath are kneaded, rolled, and manipulated in a circulatory manner, proceeding from the insertion toward the origin of the muscles, from the extremities to the trunk, in the direction of the returning blood and lymphatic currents. For this purpose the same divisions of surface as for friction will be found most convenient. Beginning then with the fingers from the roots of the nails, the thumb of the manipulator will be placed on one of the fingers of the patient, and parallel to the latter, while on the opposite

25

side the index-finger will be placed at right angles to this, and between the two the finger of the patient will be compressed and malaxated, in a rotary manner, at the rate of seventy-five to one hundred and fifty per minute. The dorsal and palmar surfaces will of course receive special attention, while the lateral aspects will come in for a secondary share. If the manipulator be sufficiently expert he can work with both hands on this small surface with the same rapidity as with one. Each finger and thumb will be taken in turn, and the manipulations extended over the metacarpal and carpal bones as far as the wrist-joint, and finally the palm of the hand by stretching the tissues vigorously away from the median line. Each part included in a single grasp may receive three or four manipulations before proceeding onward to the adjacent region. The advance upon this should be such as to allow the finger and thumb to overlap one half of what has just been worked upon. Advance and review should thus be systematically carried on, and this is of general application to all the other tissues that can be *masséed*. The force used here and elsewhere must be carefully graduated so as to allow the patient's tissues to glide freely upon each other; for, if too great, the movement will be frustrated by the compression and perhaps bruising of the tissues; if too light, the operators fingers will slip; and, if gliding with strong compression be used, the skin will be chafed. To avoid this last objection various greasy substances have been employed, so that ignorant would-be masseurs may rub without injuring the skin. When the skin is cold and dry, and the tissues in general are insufficiently nourished, as well as in certain fevers and other morbid conditions, there can be no doubt of the value of inunction; but no special skill is

27

required in order to do this, and there is no need of calling it massage unless it be to please the fancy of the patient.

The feet maybe dealt with in the same manner as the hands, using the ends of the fingers to work longitudinally between the metatarsal as well as between the metacarpal bones. Upon the arms and legs, and indeed upon all the rest of the body, both hands can be used to better advantage than where the surfaces are small. Each group of muscles should be systematically worked upon, and for this purpose one hand can usually be placed opposite to the other and in advance of it, so that two groups of muscles may be manipulated at the same time. When the circumference of the limb is not great, the fingers of one hand will partly reach on to the territory of the other, while grasping, circulatory, spiral manipulations are made, one hand contracting as the other relaxes, the greatest extension of the tissues being upward and laterally, and on the fore-arms and legs away from the median line. Subcutaneous bony surfaces, as those of the tibia and ulna, incidentally get sufficient attention while manipulating their adjacent muscles, for, if both be included in a vigorous grasp, unnecessary discomfort results. Care should be taken not to place the fingers and thumb of one hand too near those of the other, for by so doing their movements would be cramped. The elasticity, or want of it, in the patient's tissues, should be the guide, the object being to obtain their normal stretch, and in this every person is a law to himself, the character of their tissues varying with the amount and quality of adipose, modes of life, exercise, etc. A frequent error on the part of manipulators is in attempting to stretch the tissues in opposite directions at the same time, especially at the flexures of the joints, where the skin is delicate and sensitive, and where the temptation to such procedures is greatest because easiest, the effect being a sensation of tearing of the skin. The rate of these manœuvres varies from seventy-five to one hundred and fifty with each hand per minute on the arms, from sixty to ninety on the legs, and from forty to eighty on the thighs, where more force is required on account of the larger size and density of the muscles, and the need of using sufficient force to extend beneath the strong, tense fascia lata.

On the back the direction of these efforts will be from the base of the skull downward, stretching the tissues away from the spinal column while manipulating in graceful curves at an average rate of sixty per minute with each hand. And here one hand can often be re-enforced by placing the other upon it, and thus massage may be done with all the strength the manipulator can put forth. With the ends of the fingers the muscles on each side of the spinal column can be rolled, and the supra-spinous ligament can be effectually *massèed* by transverse to-and-fro movements. The ends of the fingers and part of their palmar surface should also be placed on each side of the spinous processes, and the tissues situated between these and the transverse processes worked upon by up-and-down motions parallel to the spine, taking care to avoid the too frequent error of making pushing, jerky movements in place of smooth, uniform motions in each direction.

On the chest and abdomen the same general direction will be observed as in using friction, but the manipulation will be more gentle than on the back and limbs, for the tissues will not tolerate being so vigorously squeezed and pinched. Here the massage will consist of moderate pressure and movement with the palms of the hands, and rolling and grasping the skin and superficial fascia; and, after this, on the abdomen, steady, firm, deep kneading in the direction of the ascending, transverse, and descending colon, using for this purpose the greatest force with the heel of the hand on the side of the abdomen next the operator, and on the other side the strongest manipulations with the fingers, avoiding the frequent and disagreeable mistake of pressing at the same time on the anterior portions of the pelvis.

Before leaving this part of the subject, the writer begs leave to say something more about the common errors into which manipulators fall, even some of those who pass for being skillful. Many do not know how to do the kneading or malaxation with ease and comfort to themselves and to their patients, for, in place of working from their wrists and concentrating their energy in the muscles of their hands and fore-arms, they vigorously fix the muscles of their upper arms and shoulders, thus not only moving their own frame with every manipulation, but also that of their patients, giving to the latter a motion and sensation as if they were at sea in stormy weather. By this display of awkward and unnecessary energy, not only do they soon tire themselves, and say that they have lost magnetism by imparting it to their patients, but by the too firm compression of the patient's tissues they are not allowed to glide over each other; and hence such a way of proceeding entirely fails of the object for which it is intended. Surely, cultivation is the economy of effort.

Friction and manipulation can be used alternately, varied with rapid pinching of the skin and deeper grasping of the subcutaneous cellular tissue and muscular masses, and, when necessary, with percussion, passive, assistive, and resistive movements, finishing one convenient surface or limb before passing to another, and occupying from half an hour to an hour with all or part of these procedures. Pinching is used mainly to excite the circulation and innervation of the skin, and for this purpose it is best done rapidly at the rate of one hundred to one hundred and twenty-five per minute with each hand. To act on the subcutaneous cellular tissue, a handful of skin is grasped and rolled and stretched more slowly than by the preceding method. A deeper, momentary grasping of the muscles is often advantageous, and may be called a *mobile intermittent compression,* and this, indeed, is what the whole of massage, strictly speaking, consists of. Percussion, applicable only over muscular masses, may be done in various ways. In the relative order of their importance they are as follows:

1. With the ulnar borders of the hands and fingers.

2. The same as the first, with the fingers separated.

3. With the ends of the fingers, the tips being united on the same plane.

4. With the dorsum of the upper halves of the fingers loosely flexed.

5. With the palms of the hands.

6. With the ulnar borders of the hands tightly shut.

7. With the palms of the hands held in a concave manner, so as to compress the air while percussing.

More gentle or vigorous and rapid percussion than any of these methods afford can be done by securing India-rubber air-balls on whale-bone or steel handles. With these one gets the spring of the handles together with the rebound of the balls, and thus rapidity of motion with easily varying intensity is gained, the number of blows varying from two hundred and fifty to six hundred a minute with both.

Remedial movements have been so well described in books on the so-called "movement-cure" that little need be said of them here. It is well for those who use them to know the anatomy and physiology of the joints and their natural limits of motion. Except in the case of relaxed joints, passive motion should be pushed until there is a feeling of slight resistance to both patient and manipulator; for by this will be known that in healthy joints the ligaments, capsules, and attachments of the muscles are being acted upon. Resistive movements are such as the patient can make while the operator resists. The opposing force should be carefully and instinctively kept within the limits of the patient's strength, and this, with all these other manœuvres, should stop short of fatigue. To alternately resist flexion and extension is the *pons asinorum* of manipulators, and, in a considerable experience of teaching massage, I have found but few who could learn to do it at all. Its importance cannot be overestimated as a means of cultivating the strength of weakened muscles, while, at the same time, finding out how much they can be used. Many a patient who has recovered from an old injury is still as much incapacitated as ever, from the fact that his latent energies can only be discovered and made available in this manner.

Midway between passive and resistive movements, in the course of certain recoveries, stand assistive movements. They are but little understood and seldom used. They may be illustrated as follows: Let it be supposed that, in the absence of adhesions and irreparable injury of the nerve-centers, the deltoid has but half the strength requisite to elevate the arm. So far as any use is concerned this is the same as if there were no power of contraction left in the muscle. But, if only the other half of the impaired vigor be supplemented by the carefully graduated assistance of the operator, the required movement will take place; and, in some cases, if this be regularly persisted in, together with manipulation and percussion, more vigorous contraction will be gained, and, by-and-by, the patient will exert three fourths of the necessary strength, and later the whole movement will be done without aid; and, as strength increases, resistance can be opposed to the movement. Partial loss of motion can often be accurately estimated by holding the limb suspended in a cloth attached to a spring-balance. When the patient makes effort the limb weighs less. By means of a spring-balance resistive motion can also be estimated. Still another kind of movement may be spoken of—namely, vigorous passive motion—with a view to breaking up adhesions in and about joints, a description of which does not come within the scope of this paper. It is the secret of success and of failure of the people who call themselves "bone-setters," the methods of whom have been well studied and explained by Dr. Wharton P. Hood, of London, in his very interesting book "On Bone-Setting, so called."

A description of massage of the head and the benefits that arise from it must be left to another time.

The relative importance of the foregoing procedures has been partly indicated while describing them. According to the needs of individual cases, one or more of these will predominate or be omitted, and it is well that the advice of a physician be sought on this subject, for there would be no use in giving a patient friction the capillary circulation of whose skin was already sufficiently good; and it would be a waste of time and strength to administer passive and resistive movements to patients who were already fatigued from overwork. To rouse the dormant action of cold skin and flabby muscle, percussion will be of the first importance, and will alternate with friction and manipulation. Percussion is in massage what faradization is in electricity, and will often answer the same purpose; manipulation, or deep-kneading, is to massage what the constant current is to electricity, and the ultimate effects of each are very much alike. In "Schmidt's Jahrbücher" and elsewhere numerous instances are given in which massage has succeeded, after electricity and other means had failed. The reverse of this may be true, but as yet I have not seen any proof of it. Let us now speak of the general effects of massage, and, further on, its influence more in detail. And, first, it may be well to premise that it requires, on the part of the patient a certain amount of latent energy, if one may so call it, in order to undergo even a minimum *séance* of massage; for a patient may be so weak as to preclude the possibility of its being applied without harm resulting. In properly selected cases, instances of which are frequently seen in individuals suffering from overwork, or want of work, worry, depression of spirits, and loss of sleep, together with feeble and tardy digestion—those who cannot get or take rest, no matter how favorable the opportunity—the effects of massage are generally as follows:

41

While it is being done, and often for several hours afterward, the patients are in a blissful state of repose; they feel as if they were enjoying a long rest, or had just returned from a refreshing vacation, and not a few say that it makes optimists of them for the time being. It produces warmth, comfort, and sleep; relieves or cures constipation, muscular pains, and stiffness. At the same time it exerts a peculiarly delightful and profound effect upon the nervous system, its influence being tonic, sedative, and physiologically counter-irritant, making more blood flow through the skin and muscles, and consequently less to the brain, spinal cord, and internal organs. To those to whom exercise would be injurious, massacre affords the advantages of exercise without exertion while the subjects of it are resting, their over-taxed will and used-up nervous energy not being required to express themselves in voluntary motion. For reasons such as these, we find no less an authority than the British "Journal of Mental Sciences" (for April, 1878) recommending "massage for certain melancholies, with trophic and vaso-motor affections, and also where dementia is threatened after an attack of excitement. Under this treatment mental comfort and a sense of well-being take the place of apathy and lassitude."

Lord Bacon has quaintly remarked that "repair is procured by nourishment, and nourishment is promoted by forwarding internal *concoction,* which drives forth the nourishment, as by medicines that invigorate the principal viscera; and, secondly, by exciting the external parts to attract the nourishment, as by exercise, proper frictions, etc." Massage excites the external parts to attract and assimilate the nourishment, brought thither by an increased volume of blood, and this, at the same time, favors absorption of the natural worn-out *débris*. The different ranks of the Sandwich-Islanders are of different stature; and we are told that the chiefs, though sunk in sloth and immorality, are not diminutive and decrepit, like many of their countrymen, for the reason that they fare sumptuously, take little or no exercise, and are *lomi-lomied* after every meal, in order to. aid their digestion and promote their circulation without inducing fatigue or exhaustion. *Lomi-lomi* is thus interestingly described by Nordhoff, in his book on "Northern California, Oregon, and the Sandwich Islands": "Wherever you stop, for lunch or for the night, if there are native people near, you will be greatly refreshed by the application of *lomi-lomi*. Almost everywhere you will find someone skilled in this peculiar,

44

and, to tired muscles, delightful and refreshing treatment. To be *lomi-lomied,* you lie down upon a mat, or undress for the night, if you prefer. The less clothing you have on the more perfectly the operation can be performed. To you, thereupon, comes a stout native, with soft, fleshy hands, but a strong grip, and beginning with your head, and working down slowly over the whole body, seizes and squeezes with a quite peculiar art every tired muscle, working and kneading with indefatigable patience, until, in half an hour, whereas you were weary and worn out, you find yourself fresh, all soreness and weariness absolutely and entirely gone, and mind and body soothed to a healthful and refreshing sleep. The *lomi-lomi* is used not only by the natives, but among almost all the foreign residents; and not merely to procure relief from weariness, consequent upon over-exertion, but to cure headaches, to relieve the aching of neuralgic or rheumatic pains, and, by the luxurious, as one of the pleasures of life. I have known it to relieve violent headache in a very short time. The chiefs used to keep skillful *lomi-lomi* men in their retinues; and the late king, who was for some years too stout to take exercise, and was yet a gross feeder, had himself *lomi-lomied* after every meal, as a means of aiding his digestion. It is a device for relieving pain and weariness which seems to have no injurious reaction, and no drawback but one—it is said to fatten the subjects of it."

Dr. Weir Mitchell has successfully proved that many chronic invalids can be cured by rest and excessive feeding, made possible by means of massage and electricity. Under this combination of treatment, skillfully carried out, many become fat, strong, and well, thus illustrating the truth of Lord Bacon's remark, and the beneficial effects of the not very scientific massage of the Sandwich-Islanders. The *lomi-lomi* of the Sandwich-Islanders is only a series of intermittent squeezes proceeding toward the extremities, thus hindering the returning circulation; and this illustrates another fact—that many who have had but one kind of pinching and squeezing think it is "excellent" until they try someone who understands and can do it better; moreover, it shows that any sort of stirring up of the tissues is often better than none. In using massage, as much depends on the qualities and qualifications of the person who does it as in any other occupation. It would be wrong to leave the impression that massage is always agreeable from the first. In proportion as the muscles, superficial fascia, and skin are unnaturally tough, tense, *matted* and *hide-bound,* will the massage be disagreeable until they become soft, supple, and elastic. An appreciation of the proper consistence of the tissues and their anatomical structure is of the utmost importance for the success of this treatment.

But we must hasten to consider how massage acts locally. By upward and oval friction, with deep manipulation, the vein's and lymphatics are mechanically emptied—the blood and lymph are pushed along more quickly by the additional *vis a tergo* of the massage, and these fluids cannot return by reason of the valvular folds on the internal coats of their vessels. Thus, not only is more space created for the returning currents arising from beyond the region *masséed,* but, at the same time, a vacuum is formed, which is visible in the superficial veins of persons who are not too fat; and this is thought by some to add a new force to the more distal circulation. In this way the collateral circulation in the deeper vessels is aided and relieved, as well as the more distal stream in the capillaries and arterioles. One would naturally suppose that the circulation in the larger arteries would, in this manner, be interrupted, and such is the case. But, herein comes an additional advantage to aid the circulation, for the temporary and momentary intermittent compression causes a dilatation of the artery from an increased volume of blood above the part pressed upon, and this accumulation rushes onward with greater rapidity as soon as the pressure is removed, in consequence of the force of the heart's action and the resiliency of the arteries acting upon the accumulated volume of blood.

But the same pressure also acts upon the tissues external to the vessels, causing a more rapid resorption of natural or pathological products through the walls of the venous capillaries and lymphatics. When muscular nerves are stimulated, the vaso-dilators are influenced, and this takes place by massage, whence follows enlargement of the lumen of the vessels, so that an increased flow passes through them with greater ease and diminished pressure. When stimuli are applied to the skin, reflex vaso-motor action shows that the vaso-dilators are acted upon, hence the redness and congestion of the skin when massage is specially directed to it. It can be readily seen now that massage rouses dormant capillaries, increases the area and speed of the circulation, furthers absorption and stimulates the vaso-motor nerves, all of which are aids and not hindrances to the heart's action, as well as to nutrition in general. Seeing that more blood passes in a given time, there will be an increase in the total interchange between the blood and the tissues, and thus the total amount of work done by the circulation will be greater and the share borne by each quantity of blood less. It will not be surprising, then, to learn that in practice massage sometimes proves a valuable ally in the treatment of functional and organic diseases of the heart, for "the peripheral friction of the blood against the walls of the capillaries and small arteries not only opposes the flow of blood through them, but, working backward along the whole arterial system, has to be overcome by the heart at each systole of the left ventricle." This obstacle is in great part lessened by massage. In exercise there is alternate contraction and relaxation of voluntary muscles, and this is a powerful aid to the circulation in general; for at each contraction the vessels are emptied by compression, and the alternating relaxation allows them to fill up again. Thus each muscle or group of muscles in activity has been appropriately likened to a beating heart. In this respect the intermittent pressure of massage aids and imitates the alternate contraction and relaxation of muscles very accurately, and no better praise could be bestowed upon any therapeutical agent than the old-fashioned, haughty, supercilious way of dismissing the subject of massage as unworthy of notice by saying that it was merely a substitute for exercise. Exercise favors all the functions, and people who can exercise freely without fatigue, and who can eat and sleep well, seldom need massage. I am aware that this statement includes many neurasthenics, especially those who suffer from want of occupation.

While undergoing massage it is well for the patient to take frequent and deep inspirations, in order to favor the flow of the venous and lymphatic currents to the thorax. This, however, is often instinctively done, and with such ease that the patient feels as if freed from an immense load. From a paper by Professor H. P. Bowditch, in the "Proceedings of the American Academy of Arts and Sciences," for 1873, "On the Lymph-Spaces in Fasciæ," we learn the following valuable and interesting facts: "In experiments on animals where the flow of lymph through the thoracic duct was measured, passive movements of the limbs increased this flow in a remarkable manner. Galvanization of the muscles had a similar but less powerful effect. The lymph-spaces existing between the tendinous fibers of fasciæ and the connection of these spaces with lymphatic vessels have been described by Ludwig and others. By virtue of this structure the fasciæ play an important part in keeping up the flow of lymph through the lymphatic vessels. A piece of fascia was removed from the leg of a dog and tied over the mouth of a glass funnel, with the side next the muscles uppermost. A few drops of a colored turpentine solution were then placed upon this surface, and the fascia alternately stretched and relaxed by partially exhausting the air from the funnel and allowing it to return again. In this way the coloring matter was made to penetrate into the spaces between the fibers of the fascia and to enter the lymph-spaces on the opposite side. The same result was obtained when the coloring matter was injected between the muscles and the fascia, and the latter stretched and relaxed by passive movements of the limb. The alternate widening and narrowing of the lymph-spaces between the tendinous fibers seems, therefore, to cause absorption of the lymph from the neighboring parts as well as its onward flow into the lymphatic vessels." This function of the fascia certainly affords a partial, important, and, so far as it goes, very satisfactory explanation of the success of methods of treatment which involve passive motion, for the removal of effete matters from the tissues is favored by an increased flow of lymph.

But Nature, as one of her regular functions, is continually performing this experiment in the voluntary and involuntary movements of the muscles. The large serous cavities, such as those of the pleura and peritonæum, are now regarded as extensive lacunae in the course of the lymphatic vessels; lymph-spaces and lymphatic vessels, communicating with each other by means of small openings or stomata, have been demonstrated in these membranes, and also the communication of the lymph-spaces with the pleural and peritoneal cavities by means of intercellular openings. This has been shown by injecting either of these cavities with colored fluid, and, after killing the animal, examining the course of absorption of the fluid under the microscope. In the movements of respiration, alternate expansion and contraction of the chest-walls, with descent and ascent of the diaphragm, we have a continual pump-like action of absorption and onward expulsion in the lymph-spaces and lymphatic vessels of the pleura and peritonæum. But we must not forget that the capillary blood-vessels are similarly influenced, nor should we fail to remember that osmosis may also play a very important part, and that this, too, can be increased by artificial pressure. We can now understand why the kings of the Sandwich Islands should be *lomi-lomied* after every meal in order to aid their digestion, for the externally applied pressure over the abdomen would force the contents of the lacteals, or lymphatics of the small intestine, onward, at the same time aiding them in their absorption of digestive products.

Professor von Mosengeil, of Bonn, has made some interesting and useful experiments by injecting the cavities of corresponding joints of rabbits with Indian ink, and in this way proving that resorption takes place from these cavities by means of lymph-spaces and stomata, communicating with lymphatic vessels, and through these with lymphatic glands. With each rabbit he *masséed* one of the joints and left the corresponding joint untouched. The swelling that arose from the injection always disappeared rapidly under massage, and, upon examination of the *masséed* joint, it was found emptied for the most part of its colored contents. Even when the examination was made shortly after the injection and the use of massage, there was proportionately little ink found in the joint, part of it was found upon the synovial membrane; and upon microscopic examination it was seen that the greatest part had been forced into, and had penetrated through, the synovial membrane, and the darkened lymphatics could be seen with the unaided eye from the injected joint to the lymphatic glands, and these latter were black from the absorption of the ink. Upon examination of the injected joint-cavities that had not been *masséed,* the ink was still found in the joint mixed with the synovia in a smeary mass, and it had not even penetrated into the tissue of the synovial membrane. With the removal of the effusion by the use of massage, Von Mosengeil always succeeded in improving the stiffness, and in obtaining the same appearances in the lymphatics.

From clinical experience in the use of massage in joint affections, such results as those obtained by Von Mosengeil might have been with safety predicted. A consideration of the mode of application of massage in joint injuries and affections, and its relations to mechanical support, rest, and exercise, would far exceed the limits of this paper. Scandinavian, German, and French army-surgeons, who with their own hands have used massage the most in joint maladies, have accumulated respectable and trustworthy statistics showing its great value in such cases. At the same time they have not forgotten to tabulate their failures. The result of their experience in recent joint injuries admitting of the application of massage is thus formulated: "It will simultaneously further and increase resorption, accelerate the circulation, relieve pain, and reduce elevated temperature" I have illustrated this by a report of over three hundred cases, the details of which may be found in the "New York Medical Record," No. 353. The "Nouveau Dictionnaire de Médecine" clearly expresses the action of massage in the following words: "Massage augments interstitial absorption not only by the *sur-activité* impressed upon the returning circulation, but also by dividing to infinity pathological and normal products accumulated in the muscular interstices and meshes of the cellular tissue. The dissemination of these products multiplies their points of contact with the walls of the veins and lymphatics, whence result their imbibition and diffusion into the general circulation."

But, discuss any therapeutical agent as we may, there is something still peculiar to each that evades expression by tongue or pen. Of what use is it to describe odors, tastes, sensations, sights, and sounds? They can only be comprehended by smelling, tasting, feeling, seeing, and hearing. Just so with the peculiar calm, soothing, restful, light feeling that so often results from massage, which cannot be understood until experienced. It doubtless arises to a great extent from the pressure of natural worn-out *débris* being speedily removed from off terminal nerve-filaments. Furthermore, massage excites and awakens the *muscular sense* in an agreeable and beneficial manner such as nothing else does, and we know that the state of our muscles indicates and often determines our feeling of health and vigor, or of weariness and feebleness. To many minds a more satisfactory way of explaining the phenomena produced by massage would be by saying that they all occur in consequence of "magnetism," by which they have an indefinite understanding that this is some sort of imperceptible, ethereal fluid passing from one person to another. Such an explanation is low, gross, and vulgar, and it is erroneously used as a synonym for personal influence by people who do not know the proper scientific meaning of magnetism. Those who claim to have a vast stock of "magnetism" are like those who talk much of their bravery—sensible people find them devoid of either.

The Action of Massage upon the Muscles

That "science follows art with limping strides," as so well expressed by an able physician, is perhaps nowhere oftener seen than in the various branches of the practice of medicine. Experience has taught us from time immemorial the value of massage as a nerve and muscle tonic, and, like all good things, the possibility of its overuse. But the recent experiments of Prof. Arnaldo Maggiora, of the University of Turin, so clearly and beautifully detailed in the *Archives Italiennes de Biologie* (tome xii, page 225), have demonstrated that this matter can be brought into the sunny light of exact science and away from the somber shades of quackery, where it has been so long relegated by the vast majority of the medical profession. Zabludowski, it is true, had in part prepared the way for this by showing that when after fatigue from a definite amount of work a rest of fifteen minutes was insufficient to restore the tired muscles to their former vigor, after massage for five minutes they were capable of doing as much work as before, and after massage for fifteen minutes they could do twice as much work as at first.

Prof. Maggiora endeavored to ascertain:

1. The action of massage upon muscles in a state of repose. For this purpose the fatigue curves of the right and left middle fingers in maximum voluntary flexion every two seconds with a weight of three kilogrammes (6·6 pounds) were taken at 8 and 11 A. M., at 2 and 5 P. M., and the following day the fatigue curves of the same muscles with the same weight and rhythm were taken after mixed massage (friction, percussion, and kneading) for three minutes at the same hours of the day. The

average result showed that the muscles did almost twice as much work after massage as they did before. The average of the work without massage was 4·352 kilogrammes for the left middle finger, but after massage of the finger and forearm the average was 8·019 kilogrammes before extreme fatigue stopped further contractions. An analogous series of experiments was next made in which the electrical current was employed to tire the muscles by applying it directly to them, and also to the median nerve. The results without and with massage were similar to the first series, and showed that it takes much longer to fatigue the muscles by contraction from electrical irritation after massage than before.

2. The next series of experiments were undertaken with a view to determine whether the beneficial effects of mixed massage (friction, percussion, and kneading) increased in proportion to the duration of its application. At 8 A. M. the normal fatigue curve was taken, then every two hours and a quarter after this the curve was taken, having been preceded by two, five, ten, and fifteen minutes of massage of the right and left middle fingers and their corresponding muscles in the forearm. Ten fatigue tracings were thus taken, and the result showed that with five minutes of massage all the useful effect that could be produced was obtained. When the massage was continued longer, for ten or fifteen minutes, there were but slight variations in the amount of work above and below that after five minutes. Similar experiments were made in which electricity was used to tire the muscles in place of voluntary flexion, and the same result was obtained.

3. The object of the next series of experiments was to ascertain the effects of the principal maneuvers of massage—friction, percussion, and *pétrissage,* or kneading. The mode of procedure was as before: first, the normal fatigue tracing was taken; then at regular intervals during the day, every two hours, the fatigue curve was inscribed after five minutes of friction or *effleurage,* after five minutes of percussion, after five minutes of *pétrissage,* and finally after five minutes of friction, percussion, and petrissage alternating. The results showed that there was very little difference in the work that could be accomplished after five minutes of friction as compared with five minutes of percussion. But there was a great increase in the number and strength of the contractions after *pétrissage.* The best effect, however, was obtained after the alternations of all three. (It would be interesting to reproduce the tables and tracings if space allowed.) Like results were obtained when the contractions were produced by electricity applied to the median nerve or to the muscles directly, and the friction, percussion, and *pétrissage* employed separately and alternately.

4. The effects of massage upon muscles weakened from various causes were also studied in the same exact manner by Dr. Maggiora. Upon muscles weakened from fasting the effect of massage was to restore them temporarily, so that they gave normal tracings of fatigue; and the same result was obtained when the electric current in place of the will was used to tire the muscles.

5. As the result of general fatigue, the muscles of the hand were also tried in an indirect manner. Prof. Maggiora, after a walk of ten miles, to which he was not accustomed, took a tracing of the fatigue curves of the right and left middle fingers as before, and found that they were only capable of doing one fourth as much work as when he was rested. After

massage for ten minutes they were so much temporarily rested that they did nearly a normal amount of work and gave nearly a normal tracing. The work probably would have been equal to normal had it not been for the superadded fatigue of taking the fatigue tracing half an hour before the massage; for it has been found that the muscles of the middle finger when tired by contractions with three kilogrammes every two seconds require about two hours' rest in order to give normal fatigue tracings every two hours during the day.

6. The effect of massage upon muscles weakened by loss of sleep was also inspected. In muscular fatigue from fasting rest alone does not restore them, and in fatigue from wakefulness nourishment alone affords no appreciable relief. After the loss of a night's sleep the fatigue curve was taken and found to be very small, but after ten minutes of massage it was temporarily restored to a natural curve, which could not be obtained on previous occasions by rest nor by nerve tonics alone.

7. Intense and prolonged intellectual work produces a state of general lassitude. After the final examination of twenty medical students, which lasted for five hours. Prof. Maggiora was much exhausted. He then took a fatigue curve of flexion of the middle fingers of both hands. This was only about one fifth normal. Half an hour later, after ten minutes of massage, the number of contractions was little less than natural, and might have reached natural-but for the fatigue induced by the preceding experiment.

8. After a slight attack of fever of ten hours' duration the muscles were weak the whole of the following day, but after massage the aptitude for work was increased so that the

contractions of the fingers gave almost a natural tracing of fatigue.

9. The effect of massage upon anæmic muscles was most interesting. Dr. Maggiora demonstrated that anemia for a short time—from three to five minutes—produces phenomena in muscles similar to fatigue; or, in other words, lessens their vigor and resistance to work. Compression of his brachial artery was made for three minutes, and at the end of this time, while the compression was still maintained, a fatigue tracing was taken and found to be very small, the finger contracting only eleven times. Two hours later the brachial artery was again compressed for three minutes, and at the same time the forearm was subjected to massage. At the end of three minutes, the anæmia being kept up, another tracing was taken, and the muscles contracted but nine times, when prevented by fatigue from doing more. Massage has, therefore, no effect upon muscles thus rendered so completely ansemic in the way of increasing their capability for work.

This experiment was made with a weight of one kilogramme (2·2 pounds) and contractions every two seconds. It was found that in a natural condition the middle finger could thus contract two hundred and sixty-five times without any fatigue.

In comparing this last experiment with the preceding ones it is found that the effect of massage consists essentially in reawakening the phenomena of the local circulation, in bringing to the muscles a greater quantity of material necessary for their contraction, and in removing the retrograde products of muscular work.

SUMMARIZE:

—1. Massage, when applied upon a muscle in a state of repose, increases its resistance to work and modifies its fatigue curve by retarding the manifestation thereof.

2. The beneficial effect of massage is within certain limits in proportion to the duration of its application. Beyond these limits there is not obtained any further increase in the production of mechanical work.

3. Massage can hinder in muscles the accumulated effects of fatigue proceeding from the effects of work when not sufficient intervals of rest have been allowed.

4. The various manœuvers of massage act with different intensity upon the aptitude of muscles for work. Percussion and friction are inferior to *pétrissage* and to mixed massage.

5. In muscles weakened by fasting we can, by means of massage, notably ameliorate their resistance to work.

6. Upon muscles fatigued or weakened by a cause which acts upon the whole muscular system, such as prolonged walking, loss of sleep, loss of food, excessive intellectual work, etc., massage exerts a restorative influence which brings back to them their power of doing a natural amount of work.

7. The beneficial effects of massage upon the phenomena of muscular work are no longer produced when it is applied upon a muscle in which the circulation of blood has been suppressed.

Massage in Sprains, Bruises, and Dislocations

In the Life and Letters of Mr. George P. Marsh, Volume I, page 219, is the following account of the brilliant success of the treatment of two sprains by a wild Arab: "There seemed, however, small chance that the proposed journey to Sinai, Petra, Jerusalem, etc., could be carried out. The season was already far advanced for desert travel; Mr. Marsh had seriously sprained his ankle at Karnac while carrying his wife through the great temple, and could not now walk without the assistance of two persons; and Miss Paine had been suffering from a somewhat similar sprain even before leaving Constantinople, and had profited little by the surgical skill of the Pranks at that place or in Egypt. The dragoman, though it was clearly for his interest that the journey should be made, admitted the impossibility of it under these circumstances, and gravely proposed that the two sprains should be cured at once by an Arab doctor of his own acquaintance. He entreated so earnestly and with such apparent confidence in his miracle-worker that a consultation was held with some of the oldest and most intelligent of the Frankish residents at Cairo, and, though no one would exactly take the responsibility of advising it, every one said that the evidence of these immediate cures was such that he should certainly try the experiment in his own case. Some, indeed, had tried it with entire success, and no one thought any harm could come of it.

"These considerations, added to an intense desire to see more of the mysterious East, decided the lame patients to call in the 'radoubeur.' So, the second morning after their installment in their hotel, Achmet presented himself, bringing with him the most extraordinary creature that can be well imagined. He was scarce five feet in height, and was clad in a single garment of blue cotton fastened about the waist with a leather belt. His old, withered face was lighted up by one eye only, and that seemed but half open, while nothing about his person would have led one to believe that the waters of the broad Nile were within reach. There was an unmistakable look of mortification on the part of those who had consented to summon this Aesculapius, but there was no help for it now. At this moment a visitor was announced to Mr. Marsh, and the lady therefore was the first to prove the wild man's skill. He examined the injured foot, placed it in warm water, dipped his own fingers in olive oil, and rubbed and pressed the foot very gently for about twenty minutes. He then carefully dried it and bade his patient walk. She hesitated, having suffered so much and so long from every effort of that kind; but an imperative ' *Imsheh, Imsheh*,' decided her. She placed her foot firmly on the floor and took a step, another and another, and still no pain. In a few minutes she was in the street, and, after strolling some hours among the bazaars of the city, returned without the least feeling of discomfort. The cure was perfect and permanent.

"In the meantime Mr. Marsh had passed through a more severe ordeal at the hands of the magician. His foot and ankle, which were both badly swollen and discolored, were very sensitive to the manipulation, and especially to the energetic pulling which in this case was a part of the treatment, and at the end of three quarters of an hour he was well-nigh exhausted by the pain. But then, on looking at his foot, he was surprised to find that the swelling had disappeared, the color was almost entirely natural, and the shoe and stocking, which had been laid aside for almost two weeks, were put on with perfect ease. He was then directed to walk, which to his amazement he found he could do without the least pain; and the only unpleasant sensation he experienced afterward was a slight stiffness for the first day or two, which, however, did not in the least interfere with walking. After this, preparations for forty days' wandering in the desert were made as rapidly as possible."

Making allowance for the enchantment that distance always lends, there is little doubt that these two injuries were much benefited by the manipulations of the wild Arab. But it is very evident that he hurt his second patient much more than there was any need of. It would, indeed, be strange if the teachings of science did not enable us to improve on the methods of blind instinct. And though science often follows art with limping strides, yet here we can say that science has caught up with art and together they work for the rapid amelioration of disabled joints. No sane person would think of having massage applied immediately to the seat of a sprain, but many imagine that this is what the masseur will do, and hence deprive themselves of the early benefit that might be got from this method of treatment, which quickly relieves the pain, the heat, and the swelling, removes the pressure from terminal nerve filaments, and prevents the parts from sticking together. No two masseurs are alike by nature nor in skill, tact, and education, and the one who knows his anatomy and physiology well, when called to a recent acute sprain, will not begin at once to masser the injured joint, but at a distance above it on the healthy tissues by gentle stroking or effleurage toward the heart, gradually proceeding nearer and nearer to the painful place. This has a soothing effect and pushes the flow along in the veins and lymphatics, making more space in them for the returning currents coming from beyond and carrying away the fluids that have leaked out of the vessels. The same should be done on the part of the limb beyond the joint, for the circulation is hindered both in going out and coming in by reason of the swelling.

Next, the masseur who knows his business will begin again at a safe distance above the injured joint, and use deep rubbing, kneading, or massage properly so called, one hand contracting as the other relaxes, alternately making circular grasps, with the greatest pressure upward, and this should be done on the parts above and below the seat of sprain. By this procedure the effects of the previous stroking or effleurage are much enhanced an analgesic or agreeably benumbing effect is produced upon the nerves which extend to the painful place, and the retarded circulation is pushed along more vigorously, making room in the vessels for the swelling, the effusion, the dammed embargo caused by the landslide of blood and lymph that is inundating the surrounding territory with exudates farther up the stream to float off, and preparing the way for the next step in treatment. At the end of fifteen or twenty minutes of this manner of working, gentle, firm pressure can be made immediately over the swollen and but recently very tender parts, which in a few seconds can have circular motion, with the greatest push upward added to it; and this, if sufficient tact be .used, will in all probability not hurt but be positively agreeable. By this the swelling is spread over greater space, pressed out of the tissues as water is out of a sponge, and brought into more points of contact with the veins and lymphatics by which they are absorbed and carried off; the same pressure that causes the dislodgment of stagnating fluids also aiding absorption by pressing them into the small vessels. Then a snug, well-fitting bandage should be applied, which may exhibit the bungling of a tyro or the skill acquired by twenty years' practice. Under this plan of treatment, used twice a day, the comfort produced and the speed of recovery would scarcely be believed unless experienced by one who had had a similar injury treated in the regular orthodox way, with absolute rest and immobility, by means of fixed dressings.

Some years ago I published the results of massage in more than seven hundred cases of sprains, joint contusions, and distortions of all degrees of severity, treated by many different observers, most of whom were French,

German, and Scandinavian army surgeons, in order to confirm the experience obtained in some of my own cases. The invariable result of each and all was that such injuries thus treated got well in one third of the time that similar cases did under the usual method of absolute rest and fixation, and with less tendency to subsequent weakness, pain, and stiffness. Experience teaches that the sooner after a sprain massage is begun, the quicker is the recovery. In Germany the military authorities now require a semiannual report from their surgeons upon the results of massage in injuries of joints; and the statistics of Gasener, Starke, Korner, and others clearly show the rapid results of this method, and the economy of time to the soldier. I fear it will be a long time before many of the physicians and surgeons in the United States will condescend to try their hands at massage; indeed, most physicians adopt, prescribe, or tolerate massage in the same way that Constantine the Great embraced Christianity — more from policy than conviction.

The orthodox treatment of absolute immobility alone in these cases has little else to support it than the dogmatism of centuries, from which it is almost impossible for a surgeon to free himself, unless he has been the unfortunate victim of a sprain, and had it treated with massage. Supposing a prize of ten thousand dollars were offered for the quickest way to make a well joint stiff, what more effectual means could be resorted to than first to give it a wrench or sprain, and then do it up in a fixed dressing, so that the resulting inflammation would have an opportunity of producing adhesion of the parts? And this is the prevailing treatment of sprains. The same plan of treatment is employed for the purpose of closing up holes in other parts of the body—namely, that of exciting adhesive inflammation; and, unfortunately, it sometimes closes the cavity of a joint also.

It would seem as if we had sufficient proof of the beneficial effects of massage in injuries and affections of joints in human beings, without intentionally inflicting similar injuries on animals in order to treat them by massage, and study the effects of this upon them. However, much interesting and confirmatory evidence has resulted from such experiments, and the effects produced are no longer left in the realm of theory, but brought into the sunny light of science and ocular demonstration. The mind of man may be prepossessed in favor of massage, and this would help recovery; of animals it cannot be, unless they had had massage before for a similar hurt. Animals that have been treated by massage can be killed and the effects studied and compared with similar injuries in other joints of the same animal that have not had massage. Von Mosengeil, Professor of Surgery at Bonn, injected corresponding joints of rabbits with Indian ink. With each rabbit he *masséed* one of the joints at regular intervals, and left the same joint in the other limb untouched. The swelling and stiffness caused by the injection rapidly disappeared under massage, and on examination of the *masséed* joint after the animal was killed it was found empty of its colored contents. Even when the examination was made shortly after the injection and the use of massage, there was scarcely any ink found in the joint; part of it was found upon the synovial membrane, and upon microscopical examination it was seen that the greatest part of it had been forced into and penetrated through the synovial membrane. The darkened lymphatics could even be seen with the unaided eye extending from the injected joint to the lymphatic glands in the groin or axilla, and these latter were also black from the absorption of the ink. Upon examination of the joint cavities that had not been *masséed*, the ink was found in the joint, mixed with the synovia, forming a smeary mass, and it had not even penetrated the tissue of the synovial membrane. The same results were uniformly obtained in all the experiments, showing that absorption takes place from joint cavities by means of lymph spaces and small openings communicating with lymphatic vessels, and through these with lymphatic glands.

But by far the most interesting experiments yet performed to elucidate the effects of massage on joints, muscles, and nerves are those described at length in the Archives generates de Medecine for 1891 and 1892.

Having obtained excellent results from massage in bruises of joints and muscles, in sprains and dislocations, and also in fractures, some of which were *masséed* from the commencement of the injury when there was no displacement, and others where there was displacement, after a fixed dressing had been applied as short a time as possible to keep the parts in place, M. Castex sought further opportunities to study more exactly the results of these injuries by intentionally producing them in corresponding places in two limbs of dogs, masseing the seat of one of these injuries and letting the other alone, and after five or six months killing the animals and examining the tissues that had been hurt under the microscope. He always chose the more injured limb for treatment and the other had no massage, but was left to the natural evolutions of the injuries. The effects, immediate, consecutive, and remote, were carefully noted by experts in laboratory work, who were not told which leg had been *masséed*. The experiments were done in the laboratory of Prof. Richet. The massage was done either immediately or very soon after the injuries— even in the case of the dislocations, as soon as they were set—and always with marked relief to the pain, swelling, and stiffness; so much, indeed, that after a few massages of five or ten minutes each of frictions and petrissage once a day, the dog had full use of the leg that had been *masséed*, whereas the leg that had not been *masséed* remained swollen, stiff, and painful for a long time, and in some did not recover at all. It is but fair to state that, no matter how severely-some of the dogs were injured, especially the shepherd dogs, they did not seem to mind it at all after it was over, running about as if nothing had happened as soon as they were set at liberty. These were not chosen for massage. The details are amazingly interesting, but space forbids mention of more than one of the experiments, which may be taken as a fair sample.

The two shoulder joints of a large watchdog were dislocated by inward flexion. The head of the humerus of each was plainly visible under the skin, showing a luxation forward and inward— intracoracoid. It was easily reduced, put back in place, by traction. Five minutes of massage was at once given to the right shoulder, which seemed to afford relief, judging from the grateful way in which the animal submitted; and after this a figure-of-8 bandage was applied around both shoulders. He had massage five minutes daily to the right shoulder alone, and for the first three days he walked with difficulty. The right shoulder gradually became less painful to touch, and he stood firmer on this side. On the fourth and subsequent days all sorts of pressure upon the *masséed* shoulder were borne without discomfort; but when the other shoulder was pressed the dog growled and attempted to bite. Six days after the dislocations he supported himself well in the *masséed* limb, but held the other up, as the non-7nasseed shoulder was still swollen and painful. Both shoulders then staid in place, in spite of passive movements that might have dislocated them. On the eighth day the dog walked well with the *masséed* limb, but held the other up, as the latter was still swollen and painful, and there was crepitation in the joint. Thirteen days after the injury the dog took an occasional step with the limb that had not been *masséed*, and two months later it was in about the same condition, while he made free use of the limb that had been *masséed* in walking and running. There was then atrophy (wasting) of the muscles of the left shoulder, evident by the prominence of the bones; none, of the muscles of the right.

Testimony in favor of the early use of massage in dislocations in human beings, being careful not to move nor disturb the joint, is gradually accumulating. Not only M. Castex, but also MM. Edge, Archambaud, and others, have reported more favorable results from its application from the very first day of the injury than when it had not been used. Passive motion, I think, should not be begun until the patients find that they can make a little voluntary motion. Fifteen or twenty days of this treatment seems to be all that is necessary in mankind; and this is just about the length of time required for the repair of the rent in the capsule. In the meantime, the surrounding tissues are preserved in health and activity by means of the massage.

Soon after the swelling from the injuries to the dogs had subsided the muscles became more or less atrophied in the limb that had not been *masséed*, but not at all in the limb that had been *masséed*. At the end of five or six months the dogs were killed and the tissues examined by the microscope. The muscular tissue of the side that had not been *masséed* presented a diffuse sclerosis or hardening; the connective tissue intervening between the fibers and bundles of fibers was thickened; there were interstitial hæmorrhages, especially in the cellular tissue around the muscles; the internal and external coverings of the bundles of muscular fibers (perimysia) were infiltrated with blood, and also the fascia or covering outside of this.

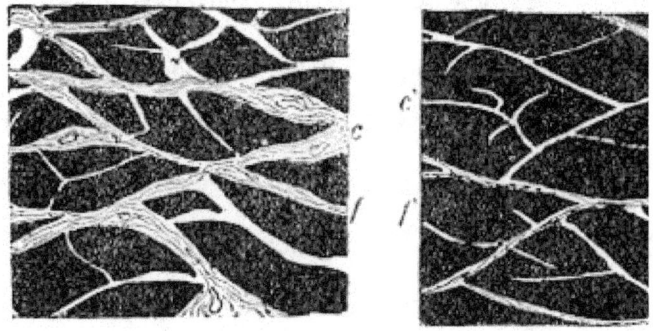

FIG. 1.—BRUISED MUSCLE WITHOUT MASSAGE. *f*, muscular fasciculus; *c*, intermuscular connective tissue.

FIG. 2.—BRUISED MUSCLE WITH MASSAGE. *f*, muscular fasciculus; *c'*, intermuscular connective tissue.

Fig. 2 shows that the natural size of the intermuscular connective tissue has been preserved, while Fig. 1 shows the intermuscular tissue thickened, and the muscular bundles thinner and compressed.

The transverse markings of the muscular fibers (striæ) were effaced in many places, while the longitudinal striation or marking,

95

which is not seen normally, was very distinct. The muscular tissue from the corresponding region that had been *masséed* was found to be normal in every particular. M. Castex has left us to surmise the appearance of the sarcolemma or covering of the individual fibers. In all probability this also was hardened, thickened, and infiltrated with blood as were the outer and larger coverings.

The blood-vessels appeared perfectly natural from the *masséed* side, but from the side that had not been *masséed* they presented a hyperplasia or thickening of their external coat.

The nerve filaments were found to be natural in the *masséed* side, while in the side that had not been *masséed* there were abundant evidences of neuritis, and perineuritis exerting destructive compression upon the nerve fibers. The perineurium, or sheath covering the bundles of nerve fibers, was at least three times as thick in the *non-masséed* side, and the connective tissue around the perineurium was also thickened with numerous new-formed cells. The small vessels in the perineurium were also the seat of a peripheral hyperplasia or thickening. The lesion of the nerves was more marked than that of the vessels.

These experiments of M. Castex give more emphasis than ever to the remarks of old Arrian in the year of our Lord 243, that "great is the advantage of rubbing to the dog, not less than to the horse, for it is good to knit and to strengthen the limbs, and it makes the hair soft and its hue glossy, and it cleanses the skin from its impurities. One should rub the back and the loins with the right hand, placing the left under the belly in order that the dog may not be hurt by being squeezed from above into a crouching position; and the ribs should be rubbed with both hands, and the buttocks as far as the feet, and the shoulder blades as well. And when they seem to have had enough, lift her up by the tail, and, having given her a stretching, let her go. And she will shake herself when let go, and show that she liked the treatment." (*Arrian Cynegeticus.*) In human beings M. Castex found that when massage was begun early or from the very first in contusions, sprains, and dislocations not only were the immediate symptoms soon relieved, but also the subsequent serious consequences that are so apt to follow these injuries—wasting, weakness, contraction, and stiffness—were prevented. But when he tried massage in old cases of muscular atrophy or wasting following injuries to joints he got no increase of muscular tissue. The stiffness was got rid of; the muscles became suppler, but they still remained thin and lacking in strength. If he had combined passive and active movements with the massage he would probably have gained growth of muscle. He found that the galvanic and faradic currents were of benefit in promoting increase of muscular tissue. Muscular contraction produced by electricity is but another form of motion.

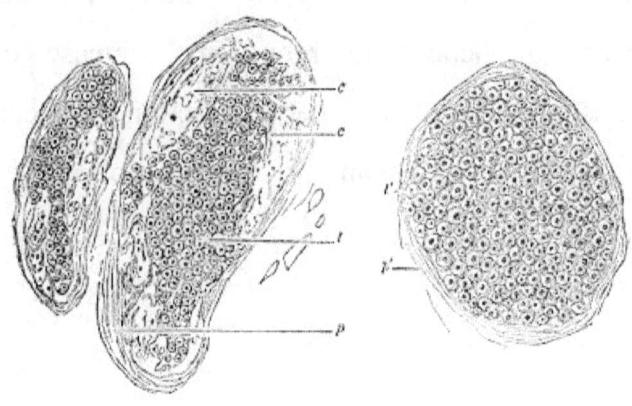

FIG. 3.—INJURED
NERVE WITHOUT
MASSAGE. *p*,
perineurium; *t*, nerve
tubes or fibers; *c c*,
new-formed
connective tissue.

FIG. 4.—INJURED
NERVE WITH
MASSAGE. *p'*,
perineurium; *t'*, nerve
tubes or fibers.

In Fig. 4 all the nerve elements arc of normal appearance, while the nerve elements from the *non-masséed* side—Fig. 3—show that the perineurium is thickened, and underneath this there are deposits of new-formed connective tissue which crowd and compress the nerve fibers.

Numerous theories as to the cause of muscular atrophy from injuries to joints have been considered and abandoned. The most probable and most generally accepted is that of reflex action. The injury to the joint starts up more or less inflammation (arthritis); the articujar nerves are irritated; this irritation is transferred to the spinal cord; the nerve centers affected act in turn upon the centrifugal nerves going to the muscles, and these determine at their peripheral ends the muscular atrophy. With a view to the elucidation of this, M. Deroche has repeated seven times, and always with the same results, experiments which were done for the first time at the College of France by MM. Raymond and Onanoff. He divided the posterior roots of the three last lumbar nerves on the left side in dogs and rabbits. After cicatrization had taken place he assured himself that numbness was complete from the thigh to the knee of the left lower limb, so that irritation of this region was not felt. The corresponding limb was left intact. An arthritis was then excited in both knees by introducing a thermo-cautery into them. No pain was felt in the left knee, but much in the right. Three months afterward the animals were killed, and in both knees the lesions of arthritis were found; hut the muscles of the thigh of the left leg were of natural size; of the right, atrophied.

Prof. Simon Duplay and M. Cazin have also made a careful study of this subject in much the same way. Under the microscope they found that the articular filaments always presented signs of inflammation; but the large nerve trunks and spinal cord showed no appreciable change, and the results of the examination of the muscles were negative except as to diminution in size. They therefore concluded that muscular atrophies consecutive to joint injuries consist of simple atrophy, and that this can only be explained by a dynamic action, a simple reflex due to irritation of the terminal nerve filaments of the articular nerves.

M. Deroche thought he found that the muscular atrophy was due to diminution of interfibrillary substance, and that there was an ascending degeneration of the posterior columns on the same side. However that may be, the inference is certainly justifiable that massage acts to prevent muscular atrophy by maintaining an influence, a movement, or something in the muscles which the spinal cord is for a time unable to impart to them; and in order to do this, it should be applied immediately or soon after the injury, for then it is more quickly aroused from the lethargy and stupor into which it has been plunged by the shock of the accident.